Nursing Skills in Nutrition, Hydration and Elimination

The body needs a constant supply of nutrients and water to survive, with water being required for the transportation of nutrients to cells and also for the transportation of waste out of the body.

This practical pocket guide focuses on what you need to know to support your patients' health and comfort. It looks at:

- The anatomy and physiology of the gastrointestinal system
- The anatomy and physiology of the renal system
- Elimination and associated skills
- Catheterisation
- Nutrition
- Hydration
- Fluid balance

This competency-based text covers relevant key concepts, anatomy and physiology, lifespan matters, assessment and nursing skills. To support your learning, it also includes learning outcomes, concept map summaries, activities, questions and scenarios with sample answers, and critical reflection thinking points.

Quick and easy to reference, this short, clinically focused guide is ideal for use on placements or for revision. It is suitable for pre-registration nurses, students on the nursing associate programme and newly qualified nurses.

Sheila Cunningham is an Associate Professor in Adult Nursing at Middlesex University, UK. She has a breadth of experience teaching nurses both pre- and post-registration and she supports mentors supporting students in practice. She is also a Middlesex University Teaching Fellow and holds a Principal Fellowship at the Higher Education Academy. She is currently programme leader for the BSc European nursing.

Tina Moore is a Senior Lecturer in Adult Nursing at Middlesex University, UK. She teaches nursing assessment, clinical skills and acute care interventions for both pre-qualifying and post-qualifying nurses. Her interests are in simulated learning approaches and Objective Structured Clinical Examination (OSCE) as a teaching and assessment method. She has authored a number of books and articles. She is also a Middlesex University Teaching Fellow.

Skills in Nursing Practice

Series editors
Tina Moore, *Middlesex University, UK*
Sheila Cunningham, *Middlesex University, UK*

This series of competency-based pocket guides covers relevant key concepts, anatomy and physiology, lifespan matters, assessment and nursing skills for good clinical practice in a range of areas from safety and protection to promoting homeostasis. To support your learning, they include learning outcomes, concept map summaries, activities, questions and scenarios with sample answers, and critical reflection thinking points.

Quick and easy to reference, these short skills-focused texts are ideal for use on placements or for revision. They are ideal for pre-registration nurses, students on the nursing associate programme and newly qualified nurses feeling in need of a little revision.

List of titles

Nursing Skills in Professional and Practice Contexts
Tina Moore and Sheila Cunningham

Nursing Skills in Safety and Protection
Sheila Cunningham and Tina Moore

Nursing Skills in Nutrition, Hydration and Elimination
Sheila Cunningham and Tina Moore

For more information about this series, please visit: www.routledge.com/Skills-in-Nursing-Practice/book-series/SNP

Nursing Skills in Nutrition, Hydration and Elimination

Sheila Cunningham and Tina Moore

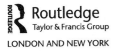

Routledge
Taylor & Francis Group

LONDON AND NEW YORK

First published 2020
by Routledge
2 Park Square, Milton Park, Abingdon, Oxon OX14 4RN

and by Routledge
52 Vanderbilt Avenue, New York, NY 10017

Routledge is an imprint of the Taylor & Francis Group, an informa business

© 2020 Sheila Cunningham and Tina Moore

British Library Cataloguing-in-Publication Data
A catalogue record for this book is available from the
British Library

Library of Congress Cataloging-in-Publication Data
A catalog record has been requested for this book

ISBN: 978-1-138-47945-6 (hbk)
ISBN: 978-1-138-47946-3 (pbk)
ISBN: 978-1-351-06570-2 (ebk)

Typeset in Stone Serif
by Wearset Ltd, Boldon, Tyne and Wear

Contents

Figures

Introduction to the Skills in Nursing Practice series

This particular book is one in a series of six *'Nursing Skills in ...'*.

Book 1 *Professional and Practice Context*
Book 2 *Protection and Safety*
Book 3 *Nutrition, Hydration and Elimination*
Book 4 *Control and Coordination*
Book 5 *Cardiorespiratory Assessment and Monitoring*
Book 6 *Mobility and Support*

These books are designed to be used in clinical practice and can be used not only for reference but also as an invaluable revision tool. There is a continuing emphasis on skills acquisition and development, particularly within nursing. This is accompanied by the increasing understanding of the necessity to effectively and efficiently integrate theory and clinical skill competence-based learning. In doing so, it ensures that nurses have the best opportunity to become 'fit to practise' and develop key employ-ability skills. Therefore, each chapter has been linked to the *Future Nurse Proficiencies* (Nursing and Midwifery Council [NMC] 2018), which will enable you, as the nurse, to map your skills development in relation to the standards set by the professional body.

The structure of each chapter within the books draws on the constructivist pedagogical approaches and assimilation theory. Each chapter has interlinking ideas and information through the use of concept maps. It is anticipated that the use of key words and connections will deepen and enhance these linkages from the concepts, drawing on general and specific aspects of a topic and will therefore promote active learning.

Concept maps are pictures or graphic representations that will help you to organise and represent knowledge of a subject. This is achieved through helping you to link, differentiate and relate concepts to each other. The concept maps begin with a main idea (or concept) and then branch out to show how that main idea can be broken down into specific topics. They can also visually represent relationships between concepts and ideas in a quick, easy-to-understand format. Concept mapping is becoming increasingly popular as a means of teaching and learning within education. The introduction of concept maps will provide a quick summary **with** additional key information of the material read in the *Clinical Skills for Nursing Practice* book. We have also included related anatomy and physiology together with lifespan matters.

The end of each chapter has questions (answers also provided) in the format of a quiz. This will help you to test your know knowledge, understanding and application of the content. There is also the opportunity for you to critically reflect on your learning using a SMART (specific, measureable, achievable, realistic and time-frame) format. From this you should then be able to clearly identify areas for future development and learning.

These pocket-size books are designed not only to help develop further your clinical skills (practice and knowledge), but also to improve your key transferrable skills, enabling them to advance your employability skills, i.e. problem solving, analytical and critical thinking, and team working. Therefore another aim for each book is to concentrate on scaffolding learning, as a result supporting, promoting and developing autonomous learning, questioning (informed) and critical thinking. The use of concept mapping allows reorganisation of information in a visual manner to promote critical thinking in the student nurse. Through concept mapping students can see how ideas/patient care needs and the interrelationships that exist promote critical thinking in relation to clinical practice.

The books within this series are not designed to be comprehensive textbooks. It is the practice companion of the *Clinical Skills for Nursing Practice*, and is designed to be used together with that book. The design of these 'pocket-size' books will enable students/readers to use them as a resource while working within and outside clinical practice.

Tina Moore and Sheila Cunningham

Introduction and overview

It is recognised that optimal physical functioning and lifestyle significantly affect our health. This is true for nutrition (undernutrition and overnutrition) as well as the maintenance of removal of waste products from these normal physiological processes. Adequate nutrition and hydration are essential for general health and wellbeing, maintaining a healthy weight and to ensure adequate growth/development in children, plus help in preventing or treating a range of conditions such as wound healing, pressure ulcers and acute kidney injury (AKI).

The maintenance of continence is also an important area of nursing and healthcare. Enabling healthy bladder and bowel care can enable patient or client independence and self-care, and salvage any anxiety or embarrassment. Healthy bladder and bowel activity can vary from person to person and from day to day. In any event what is normal for one person may not be normal for another. Patterns are key to understanding what is normal for a person and deviations from that normal such as straining to eliminate or frequent urination (or reduced) control require further exploration.

CHAPTER 1

Nutrition

Tina Moore

Overview

The importance of maintaining a healthy dietary intake and exercise has been advocated within nursing and now society for many years. Careful monitoring and promotion of adequate nutritional input are an essential part of the nurse's role to promote recovery and prevent additional problems for the patient.

Link to *Future Nurse Proficiencies* (Nursing and Midwifery Council [NMC] 2018)

Platform 4 Providing and evaluating care: specifically 4.6

Skills annexe B, part 1: Procedures for assessing people's needs for person-centred care. Specifically 2.6: accurately measure weight and height, calculate body mass index and recognise healthy ranges and clinically significant low/high readings.

Skills annexe B, part 2: Procedures for the planning, provision and management of person-centred nursing care. Specifically 5.1: observe, assess and optimise nutrition and hydration status and determine the need for intervention and support. 5.7: manage artificial nutrition and hydration using oral, enteral and parenteral routes. 5.9: manage fluid and nutritional infusion pumps and devices.

Expected knowledge

- An overview of basic food groups
- Factors affecting the individual's ability to eat a healthy diet

Introduction

As with the recording of fluid balance (next chapter), nutrition within some sectors of nursing, does not receive the amount of attention that it should and would benefit from improvements. Nutrition is essential for the functional maintenance and survival of cells. During periods of ill health, an individual's daily requirements can double. Another 'at-risk' group is the ageing population. The problem here is that the older person's nutritional requirements have not been so well defined. In addition, both lean body mass and basal metabolic rate decline with age, resulting in their energy requirement (per kilogram of body weight) also being reduced, and making this group particularly vulnerable to malnutrition. Malnutrition is the state in which there is a deficiency in energy, protein and other essential nutrients, causing adverse effects on body tissue, function and composition. Signs and symptoms of malnutrition include: weight loss that is unplanned; increased susceptibility to infections; delayed wound healing; irritability; osteoporosis; muscle loss/weakness.

Disorders that have been linked to poor nutritional intake can include: cancer, diabetes, cardiovascular and cerebrovascular disease, and osteoporosis.

Content

Nutritional – body mass index assessment	Enteral feeding	Percutaneous endoscopic gastrostomy (PEG) feeding
Total parenteral nutrition (TPN)		

Learning outcomes

- Demonstrate knowledge and understanding how to identify the importance of a balanced healthy nutritional intake
- Assess a patient's nutritional status
- Recognise the signs and symptoms of factors contributing to a deteriorating nutritional state
- Differentiate the different types of nutritional support available

Key background

Conducting a comprehensive nutritional assessment and ensuring that the patient's nutritional needs are met is very much part of the nurse's role. Nurses should work in collaboration with a nutritionist. Adequate nutrition is vital for physical and psychological wellbeing, even to the extent that the patient's quality of life can be improved.

At the time of writing the daily reference intakes for adults are: energy: 8,400 kJ/2,000 kcal; total fat: <70 g; saturates: <20 g; carbohydrate: at least 260 g; total sugars: 90 g; protein: 50 g; salt: <6 g. This is elaborated on in the 'Eat Well Guide' which is an interactive web resource that explains, in great detail, the type of food and food combinations that can be taken to maintain a healthy diet. The 'Eat Well Guide' can be found AT www.nhs.uk/live-well/eat-well/the-eatwell-guide.

Children have different nutritional needs. Between the ages of two and five, children should gradually move to eating the same foods as the rest of the family in the proportions shown in the 'Eat Well Guide'. Therefore this guide does not apply to under two year olds. It has long been recognised that primarily breast milk (for at least six months) is the most valuable feed to promote the growth, development and overall health of babies, because breast milk contains the nutrients that babies require, in addition to antibodies to help boost their immunity and protect them from various common childhood infections. The World Health Organization (WHO 2017) recommends that infants should receive complementary foods with continued breastfeeding up to two years of age or beyond.

To help eat healthily many food packages are now colour coded. The red, amber and green colour coding on the front of food packs helps to quickly assess whether a food is high (red), medium (amber) or low (green) in fat, saturated fat, sugars or salt.

There are a number of routes and devices that can support meeting the needs of individuals during their period of ill health.

NUTRITIONAL/BMI ASSESSMENT

Assessment

- Physical appearance: do they appear emaciated or are they wearing very loose clothing?
- Any influences on food intake, e.g. recent bereavement, stress?
- Weight
- Height
- BMI (body mass index)
- Observation of skin turgor
- Presence of skin breakdown or pressure sores: could be due to a compromised immune system, possible vitamin deficiency and/or undernourishment
- Mobility: can be weakened/reduced due to a reduction in muscle mass
- Religious influences
- Personal preferences
- Current weaning practices for the child
- Vital signs including a blood pressure: providing a baseline for reassessment
- Oral cavity
- Signs of dysphagia
- Any gastro-intestinal problems, e.g. vomiting, nausea, diarrhoea, constipation

Anthropometric measurements
One of the most important measurements here is weight, which can indicate the severity of malnutrition. Some diseases can cause weight loss so this needs to be considered, e.g. cancer, oedema, cachexia.

Factors contributing to a deteriorating nutritional state

- A decreased oral intake due to nausea/vomiting/inability to swallow (from surgery, stroke, coma, obstruction or even an impaired mental state).
- Periods of hospitalisation resulting in anxiety from a change of environment, a variance in mealtimes, unusual foods and being kept 'nil by mouth'.
- The body's altered requirements, i.e. where the individual has impaired digestion and absorption, or the increased requirement from burns, fever, and fractures.
- Drug therapy and its variety of side effects.
- Lack of availability of skilled staff to assist individuals with eating.

A nutritional assessment is a mandatory requirement for all patients admitted to hospital (NICE 2006) and involves vulnerable patients for whom an admission to hospital can be quite upsetting. This would include individuals with learning difficulties, impaired mental health status, children and older people.

Toddlers require a higher amount of fat and a lower amount of fibre as part of a healthy diet compared to children over the age of five and adults. Ideally, the toddler's diet should consist of three meals and two or three nutritious snacks in a day.

Children who are all require their weight to be monitored more frequently as they can lose weight a faster rate. It is recommended that children over 2 years should be weighed at least weekly. In addition, health care professionals should take care to look at the previous weights and heights of the child. Attention in the under 5 year age group should be paid to their centile charts, in their 'red' books (personal child health record).

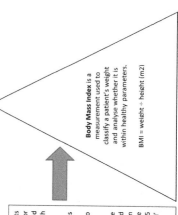

Body Mass Index is a measurement used to classify a patient's weight and analyse whether it is within healthy parameters.

BMI = weight ÷ height (m2)

FIGURE 1.1 Nutritional – body mass index assessment

ENTERAL FEEDING

Pre-procedure

- Patient is carefully assessed regarding the suitability of this approach. Assess the status of both nostrils.
- Correct positioning of the NG tube has to be confirmed before any fluid allowed to be inserted. This is done by either pH testing or x-ray.
- pH testing should be the first line method of testing tube position, with a pH of 1–5.5 being the safe range.
- Document the results.
- When there is no aspirate or the pH strip fails to reveal results, a chest x-ray should be done.

Procedure

- Explain procedure and gain consent. For the child, consider the use of play/co-operation from relatives as this can be very distressing for the child.
- Agree a method whereby the patient can indicate when to stop.
- Wash and dry hands
- Sit patient in a semi-Fowler or Fowler position (uncles contraindicated), keep head supported by pillows.
- Put on gloves, all aspects of the insertion procedure should follow the aseptic non touch technique (ANTT).
- Measure the distance of the tube to be inserted – measuring from the patient's earlobe to the bridge of the nose, then an additional measurement from the bridge of the nose to the bottom of the xiphisternum. For neonates: measure from the nose to ear and then to the halfway point between xiphisternum and umbilicus. Both points of measurement together are the required distance.
- Pass the tube through the nose and down the nasopharynx and oropharynx and further down the oesophagus. If the patient is able to drink sips, this may help with a smoother passage. Small children may need to be swaddled.
- If there are signs of breathlessness or coughing, remove the tube immediately.
- Any resistance – do NOT use force.
- Once passed, aspirate a small amount of fluid.
- Conduct pH testing.
- Once confirmed position is correct – tape the tube to patient's face/nose.
- Take off gloves and wash hands.
- Documentation.

Enteral feeding

Enteral feeding via a nasogastric tube is designed to provide a relatively short-term solution for nutritional problems and is designed for a period of 2–4 weeks. Nasogastric tubes can be inserted by nurses but ONLY with patients who are assessed as having adequate 'cough and gag' reflexes to prevent aspiration. If in doubt, patients can be referred to a speech and language therapist for assessment. For patients who do not have adequate cough or gag reflexes (e.g. someone who is unconscious), a doctor/anaesthetist will perform this skill.

Enteral feeding can be provided through nasogastric; nasojejunal; gastrostomy; jejunostomy tubes. This should not be used as a long-term solution to feeding.

In children, this is the most common route for feeding.

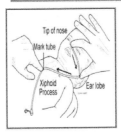 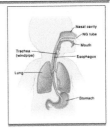

Equipment required for passing a nasogastric tube

1× Pair of gloves
Appropriate sized fine-bore nasogastric tube (child/adult)
Introducer (for tube if required)
Receiver
20ml (for child), 50ml (for adult) enteral syringe
Sterile water
pH testing paper and reference chart
Hypoallergenic tape to secure the tube in place
Glass of clean water

Aspirating a nasogastric tube

A nasogastric tube can also be used for the draining of stomach contents. This can be done via a pump, intermittent (syringe) or gravity. A wide-bore tube is used initially to enable aspiration of the tube 4-hourly (to determine pH). For longer-term feeding, a thin-bore tube should replace the original tube.

Patients should never lay flat as this can cause aspiration of stomach contents into the lung.

Record on fluid balance chart.

Dangers of enteral feeding

Patients should be monitored for signs of:
- Pulmonary aspiration
- Nausea and vomiting
- Diarrhoea
- Tube blockage
- Nasal trauma
- Over feeding

FIGURE 1.2 Enteral feeding

PERCUTANEOUS ENDOSCOPIC GASTROSTOMY TUBE (PEG)

This is used for long-term feeding where there has been a gastrostomy made.

This method of enteral feeding is safer, as the tube has a reduced risk of aspiration or dislodgement. It can be used in instances where the patient is unable to consume nutrients; impaired swallowing or sucking; unable to consume nutrients; facial, oesophageal abnormalities; anorexia related to chronic illness. Generally, all patients who have not been eating for over three days should be considered for nutritional support.

A tract is made into the stomach via endoscopy under local anaesthetic and a feeding tube is inserted. It is held in place by an external fixation device and a soft plastic bumper internally.

A dietician provides advice and information on assessment of nutritional status, nutritional intake, nutritional requirements and advice on the most appropriate route for feeding and nutritional supplementation.

Caring for PEG

1. Explain procedure to the patient and gain consent. For the child – play may need to be initiated.
2. Wash and dry hands before and after the procedure.
3. For a newly placed gastrostomy, remove the dressing and note the wound site, e.g. signs of odour, swelling, or discharge.
4. Clean the site in a clockwise motion using aseptic non touch technique (ANTT). Use one piece of gauze in a sweeping fashion then discard in the clinical waste bag.
5. In order to prevent the tube sticking to the sides of the stoma, rotate the gastrostomy tube 360°.
6. If the gastrostomy is under three months, the pH should be to be checked prior to every use.
7. Change giving set every 24 hours.
8. The gastrostomy tube will require frequent flushing, to maintain the patency. This should also be done before and after each feed and administering medication. Ideally the tube with 20ml water (if the patient is under 1 year old then it should be 5ml cooled boiled water; children is 5–15ml water).
9. Monitor for breathlessness, coughing, regurgitation of food or vomit during feed. If any occur turn off feed immediately and escalate.
10. Patient should not have an immersive bath for two weeks but can have showers.
11. Oral hygiene.
12. Monitor bowel movement.
13. Weigh at least weekly.
14. Documentation.

Complications

- ❖ Infection (redness, swelling, heat, offensive odour)
- ❖ Increased exudate
- ❖ Bleeding
- ❖ Pain or discomfort
- ❖ Leakage around the tube from the stoma
- ❖ Leakage from the device

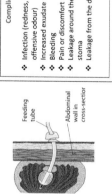

Feeding tube

Abdominal wall in cross-section

FIGURE 1.3 Percutaneous endoscopic gastrostomy (PEG) feeding

TOTAL PARENTERAL NUTRITION (TPN)

Total parenteral nutrition is used when the usual method of eating, digesting and absorbing is not possible.

Reasons for using TPN (short-term) include:
- A non-functioning gut
- Inaccessible gastro-intestinal tract
- Intestinal failure
- Patient's nutritional intake has been minimal for more than five days, or they have been 'nil by mouth' for a significant period of time
- Patient who are malnourished
- Patients with complications of treatment, e.g. chemotherapy
- Bowel obstruction

Longer-term reasons for TPN include:
- Major trauma
- Severe malabsorption
- Severe disease or damage to the intestine (in Crohns disease and short bowel syndrome)

TPN is given via either a central or a peripheral line depending on the type of TPN to be administered as well as the duration.

Close monitoring of patient's baseline observations, plus patient's urinary functioning for secretion of sodium, potassium and nitrogen.

Before commencing TPN, conduct a baseline assessment of:
- height and weight
- biochemistry: urea and electrolytes (including calcium, magnesium and phosphate)
- liver function tests
- blood glucose
- fluid balance
- temperature.

Should be undertaken and monitored throughout the infusion. In addition, urinary sodium, potassium and nitrogen should be sent for laboratory analysis to assess kidney function .

All bags of TPN are sensitive to the light, therefore when a nurse has set the infusion up and it is running the solution should be covered with a plastic bag.

Once the infusion is running it should not be disconnected for any reason. If after commencement the circuit is broken for any reason then that TPN must be discarded for safety, as it carries the risk of infection.

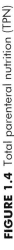

FIGURE 1.4 Total parenteral nutrition (TPN)

Activity: now test yourself

1   List four food groups (dietary requirements) and state their functions

2   State whether the following is true or false:
    It is recommended that children under age two years should eat the same as adults but purified

3   List three complications of PEG feeds

4   Which method is NOT accepted in checking that the nasogastric tube is in the correct position?

    a   pH only

    b   pH and, if no aspirate, then X-ray

    c   the 'whoosh' test

Answers

1   Four from the following list:

Carbohydrates: potatoes, bread, rice, pasta. Starchy foods are a good source of energy and the main source of a range of nutrients in our diet. As well as starch, they contain fibre, calcium, iron and B vitamins. Can put on weight if eating excessively.

Milk and dairy products: milk, yogurt, cheese. Helps with the growth of bones and teeth. Too many fats can lead to high levels of cholesterol.

Protein: beans, pulses, fish, meat. Maintains basic cell structure and growth. Can aid wound healing.

Unsaturated fats: vegetable oil, low-fat spread. Fat helps with the absorption of vitamins A, D and E. These vitamins are fat soluble, meaning that they can be absorbed only with the help of fats. Fats also help with energy. Too much can increase cholesterol.

Sugar: crisps, chocolate, fizzy drinks. Not required in our diet so can be reduced or removed. Too much can lead to weight can and disorders linked to obesity.

2   False – breast milk is strongly recommended; if not then formula milk

3   Infection (redness, swelling, heat, offensive odour)

Increased exudate

Bleeding

Pain or discomfort

Leakage around the tube from the stoma

Leakage from the device

4   The 'whoosh' test is undertaken by rapidly injecting air down a nasogastric tube while auscultating over the epigastrium and hearing a gurgling sound to indicate that it is in the stomach. No sound would indicate that the tip is placed somewhere other than the stomach. This approach is unreliable and therefore should not be used in practice.

Reflection: ask yourself

1 What do I know that I did not know before?

```
[                                                    ]
```

2 What am I confused about now?

```
[                                                    ]
```

3 What areas do I need to focus on?

```
[                                                    ]
```

4 My action plan for further learning (make objectives SMART: specific, measurable, achievable, realist and timeframe)

```
[                                                    ]
```

CHAPTER 2

Hydration and fluid balance

Tina Moore

Overview

Water is involved in every bodily function, for example circulation, digestion and elimination, regulation of body temperature. Therefore, water is one of the major requirements for survival. Unlike other deficiencies, without water life will be sustained for only a few days.

Link to *Future Nurse Proficiencies* (NMC 2018)

Platform 4 Providing and evaluating care: specifically 4.6

Skills annexe B, part 1: Procedures for assessing people's needs for person-centred care. Specifically 2.2: undertake venepuncture and cannulation and blood sampling, interpreting normal and common abnormal blood profiles and venous blood gases. 2.5: manage and interpret cardiac monitors, infusion pumps, blood glucose monitors and other monitoring devices.

Skills annexe B, part 2: Procedures for the planning, provision and management of person-centred nursing care. Specifically 5.1: observe, assess and optimise nutrition and hydration status and determine the need for intervention and support. 5.4: record fluid intake and output and identify, respond to and manage dehydration or fluid retention. 5.8: manage the administration of IV fluids. 5.9: manage fluid and nutritional infusion pumps and devices.

Expected knowledge

- Anatomy and physiology of the urinary and gastrointestinal system
- An overview of the homeostatic maintenance of fluid balance
- Principles of aseptic technique

Introduction

Water and the maintenance of adequate fluid balance are essential for sustainability. Good hydration also helps to prevent or treat certain ailments, such as constipation, urinary tract infections or kidney stones.

Yet this continues to be an area of nursing practice that is done poorly and apparently little value is placed on the assessment of the patient's fluid status and overall use of fluid balance charts within general care areas. This may stem from a lack of clear guidelines and knowledge to clarify what needs to be recorded and what impact it has on the overall care of the patient. Failure to properly recognise and respond to fluid and electrolyte disturbances in patients may have detrimental consequences. Effective fluid management relies on accurate assessment of the patient, which includes fluid balance.

Older people have very similar water requirements to those of younger adults. Estimates indicate that the older person should drink no less than 1.6 litres of water per day (Hodgkinson *et al.*, 2003). Although a survey of hospitals revealed that the actual consumption in many cases is much less (Care Quality Commission, 2011). Dehydration has been identified as a patient safety issue (Royal College of Nursing [RCN] and National Patient Safety Agency [NPSA] 2007).

Content

Introduction to fluid balance	Dehydration	Fluid overload
Electrolytes	Peripheral venous cannula (PVC)	Intravenous infusions
Starting an intravenous infusion	Delivery pumps	Blood transfusion

Learning outcomes

- Demonstrate knowledge and understanding of the importance of fluid balance and summarise how fluid balance is measured and maintained
- Assess a patient's fluid status
- Recognise the different types of delivery pumps
- Be able to prime correctly a giving set for intravenous (IV) fluid administration and safely care for a patient with an IV infusion
- Understand the principles for administering blood

Key background

Fluid and electrolyte homeostasis is maintained by the cardiovascular, renal, respiratory and gastrointestinal systems, the skin and the brain. In illness, where cardiac volume is insufficient, there is renal impairment, and selective reabsorption takes place. This results in sodium retention and excretion of potassium both inside and outside the cell (extracellular fluid compartment [ECF]) to maintain normal osmolality and blood volume. There is also movement of water between the extracellular and interstitial compartments through the process of osmosis (osmotic pressure). Loss or gain of relatively small amounts of fluid and electrolytes can influence a delicate balance in an unstable patient.

Through careful monitoring of the patient's fluid status using the skills of assessment, including an accurate fluid-balance recording, nurses are in a key position to predict, recognise and initiate prompt action in relation to issues of fluid imbalance

INTRODUCTION TO FLUID BALANCE

Homeostatic control

➤ Reduction in **renal** perfusion stimulates the release of renin by the juxtaglomerular apparatus. Renin converts angiotensinogen to angiotensin 1, further metabolised to angiotensin 11 (a vasoconstrictor and antinatriuretic hormone). Sodium is retained. Angiotensin 11 enhances sodium reabsorption.

➤ Regulation of electrolyte levels in the ECF.

➤ Regulation of acid base balance.

➤ **Atrial natriuretic peptide (ANP)**, a hormone, released from the right atrium when there is increased venous return (overload). Acts on renal system to cause diuresis (sodium and water).

➤ **Antidiuretic hormone (ADH)** released by the pituitary gland. ADH regulates the amount of water retained or excreted by the kidneys.

Functions of water

Water is an essential requirement for humans. In its absence, life can only be sustained for a few days. Total body water volume is tightly controlled with sensitive mechanisms that respond to changes in osmolality or intravascular volume.

- Maintains and regulates body temperature
- Helps maintain acid base balance
- Transports nutrients and oxygen to the cells
- Dissolves minerals and other nutrients to make them accessible to the body
- Lubricates joints, moistens tissues, i.e. in the eyes, mouth, nose
- Protects body organs and tissues (acts as an insulator and shock absorber)
- Excretion of metabolic waste products
- Helps prevent constipation

Assessment of fluid status

Assess lifestyle in relation to fluid intake – should be
Observe skin, mucosa, conjunctiva – should be moist
Skin turgor
Record temperature, pulse, blood pressure and respiratory patient's weight
Record temperature, pulse, breath sounds
Measure patient's weight
Measure fluid intake
Measure fluid output and other types of output
Measure urine output and fluid balance
Calculate overall fluid balance
Asses serum urea and electrolyte levels

Approximate daily values of fluid input and output in health

INPUTS

Oral fluid intake (~1500 ml)

Food (~500 ml)

Metabolism (~500 ml)

TOTAL – 2500 ml

OUTPUTS

Urine (~1500 ml)

Insensible loss
- sweat
- lungs
- faeces
(~1000 ml)

TOTAL – 2500 ml

Compartmentalisation of total body water in an average 70 kg man

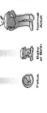

70 kg man
42 litres

Total body water

Intracellular fluid 28 litres

Extracellular fluid 14 litres

Interstitial fluid 9.5 litres

Plasma 3.5 litres

Transcellular fluid 1 litre

Transcellular fluid – secretions of the salivary glands, pancreas.

The body is divided into a number of compartments (see above). There is also a 'third space' which occurs in illness. Fluid will accumulate in areas that do not normally have fluid, or minimal amount, e.g. oedema, ascites, pleural effusion. Hypovolaemia can occur in extreme cases.

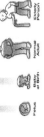

Percent of Water in the Human Body

100%   80%   70%   50%

Fetus   Baby at Birth   Normal Adult   Elderly Person

FIGURE 2.1 Introduction to fluid balance

DEHYDRATION

Types of fluid loss

Hypertonic
Body water loss, through food and fluid deficiency.

Hypotonic
Loss of fluids and electrolytes (particularly sodium). Loss also from haemorrhage, burns, peritonitis. This is more related to hypolvolaemia rather than dehydration.

Isotonic
Loss in excess of water excretion. Occurs when a disproportionate amount of free water is retained in the intracellular compartment. Can occur in diabetic ketoacidosis, disorders causing excessive gastro-intestinal loss, and excessive use of diuretics.

Dehydration is defined as the **loss of one per cent of or more of body weight (BW)**

Mild = 4 percent loss of BW

Moderate = 5–8 percent of BW

Severe = 8–10 percent of BW

(Thibodeau and Patton 2012)

Dehydration

Fluid loss of extracellular fluid occurs when water loss exceeds water intake over a period of time and the body is in a negative balance. This will lead to hypovolaemia and reduced cardiac output (diminished pre-load). Symptoms of hypovolaemia originate from reduced cardiac output, disruption of normal cellular metabolism and homeostatic mechanisms of compensation (increased heart rate, normotensive, oliguria, tachypnoea). When compensation fails then hypovolaemic shock will occur (hypotension, increasing tachycardia, poor perfusion, signs of hypoxaemia, dry skin, mouth and tongue).

Body Water
— Extracellular (33%) → Interstitial (25%), Plasma (8%)
— Intracellular (66%)

Management

❖ Treating the cause
❖ Initial monitoring, at least hourly
❖ If tolerated, oral fluids
❖ Fluid requirements in children vary depending on age and weight
❖ Isotonic saline (0.9%) for rapid volume replacement (but expands ECF and does not enter ICF)
❖ Hypotonic saline (0.45%) used with volume depletion and hypernatremia
❖ Replacing the depleted electrolytes
❖ Depending on degree of volume depletion, colloids may be used

Fluid Loss in Children

◻ Infants prone to fluid loss than adults due to:
■ A higher proportion of fluid in the EC compartment
■ Greater surface area in relation to body mass
■ Higher metabolic rate
■ Immature kidneys and immature haemostatic regulation system(buffer)
■ Greater insensible water loss
■ Inability to shiver or sweat to control temperature

Sources of fluid loss

➤ Diarrhoea
➤ Vomiting
➤ Sweating
➤ Burns
➤ Drug therapy (e.g. diuretics)

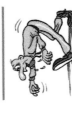

FIGURE 2.2 Dehydration

FLUID OVERLOAD

Fluid volume excess

This involves the abnormal retention of fluid and sodium. Possible causes include:

➤ Excessive sodium and/or fluid intake (e.g. overloading with fluid, over-administration of sodium (particularly intravenous), over-administration of enteral feeds/TPN

➤ Sodium and water retention (e.g. compromised regulatory mechanisms, heart failure, chronic renal failure)

➤ Fluid shift into the intravascular space (e.g. liver cirrhosis)

➤ Malnutrition, dietary (low protein intake)

Symptoms

Respiratory	Tachypnoea, signs of pulmonary oedema (productive cough, crackles, dyspnoea)
Circulatory	Increased heart rate, blood pressure, CVP and JVP, bounding pulse
Elimination	Possible increased urine output
Neurological	Headache, fatigue, irritability, confusion, seizures, coma
Oedema	Swelling – sacrum, legs feet. In children presentation tends to be face, feet and hands. Oedema – anywhere where there is tissue. Generalised (body) oedema in severe cases. Pitting oedema
Skin	Warm, moist, shiny, skin leaking fluid
General	Weight gain, generalised body oedema
Miscellaneous	Ascites, pleural effusion, abdominal distension, decreased BUN, decreased haematocrit

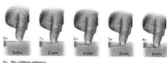

0+ No pitting oedema
1+ Mild pitting edema. 2 mm depression that disappears rapidly.
2+ Moderate pitting edema. 4 mm depression that disappears in 10–15 seconds.
3+ Moderately severe pitting edema. 6 mm depression that may last more than 1 minute.
4+ Severe pitting edema. 8 mm depression that can last more than 2 minutes.

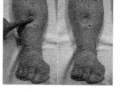

Management

- Diuretic therapy:
  moderate oedema - Thiazides (e.g. Bendrofluazide)
  severe hypervolaemia – loop diuretics (e.g. Furosemide)
  potassium sparing (e.g. amiloride)
- Monitor electrolyte levels, particularly sodium and potassium (these may need to be replaced if diuretic therapy is too aggressive)
- If able, monitor weight daily
- Sit patient in a semi-Fowler or high-Fowler position
- Limit sodium intake
- Record and monitor fluid intake, output and overall balance (aim is for a negative balance)
- Monitor vital signs, abdominal girth (if abdomen is distended)
- Ensure balanced nutrition – if malnourished, depending on severity, provide supplements or TPN
- Remove restrictive clothing, elevate swollen limb
- Compression – pressure stockings or intermittent pneumatic compression (via compression pump)

FIGURE 2.3 Fluid overload

ELECTROLYTES

Electrolytes are essential for cellular activity. Their concentration in the blood is kept within a specific range through the process of homeostasis. Changes in their levels can be life-threatening. Caution is required for those administering medication to patients with mental health disorders as certain medicines, e.g. lithium carbonate, can have severe effects for people, i.e. altering sodium levels (Gitlin 2016).

Potassium
(normal range = 3.5–5.0mmol/l)

- Closely related to reabsorption of sodium and hydrogen ions
- Major cation in the ICF compartment, maintains osmotic pressure and volume within ICF
- Essential for transmission and conduction of nerve impulses (contraction of skeletal, cardiac and smooth muscles)
- Necessary for movement of glucose into cells

Hypokalaemia (<3.5mmol/l)
Reduced potassium intake (anorexia), excessive potassium loss (diarrhoea and vomiting). May cause cardiac arrhythmias
Symptoms – weakness of respiratory muscles, leg and generalised body cramps
Treatment – Potassium replacement oral or slow IV infusion

Hyperkalaemia (>5.0mmol/l)
Increased potassium intake. Increased supply – hypercatabolic states (e.g. ACS, cardiac arrest, massive injury, infection), resulting in wide release of potassium ions from the cells into the ECF. Poor excretion due to renal failure, diabetes.
Symptoms – ECG changes, hypotension, cardiac arrest if >7.0mmol/l
Treatment – calcium gluconate or calcium chloride protects the heart, sometimes insulin and glucose

Continuous monitoring for both problems

Sodium
(normal range 135–145mmol/l)

- Sodium is widely distributed in the body, although most of it is in the ECF (maintains osmotic pressure)
- Essential for nerve impulses and muscle contractions
- Influences acid base balance; chloride and potassium levels

Hyponatraemia
Increased water intake with decreased sodium intake; overuse of diuretics; water gain in heart failure, liver cirrhosis; dilutional hyponatraemia.
Symptoms – headache, can lead to serious neurological disturbances, e.g. coma, convulsions, confusion; muscle cramps
Treatment – dependent upon the cause; if fluid loss, 0.9% saline

Hypernatraemia
Develops in response to increased ECF osmolality (water moves out of the cells, leading to cellular dehydration), overuse of sodium, severe vomiting and diarrhoea (excessive water loss)
Symptoms – convulsions, drowsiness, lethargy, confusion, coma may occur
Treatment – if overhydrated, diuretics and restricted sodium intake

Calcium
(normal range 2.1–2.6mmol/l)
Involved in building strong bones and teeth and blood clotting.

Hypocalcaemia
Paraesthesia, tetany, seizures, abdominal spasms, laryngeal spasm, irritability, decreased cardiac output, bleeding
Treatment – oral calcium and vitamin D supplements, IV calcium gluconate

Hypercalcaemia
Muscle weakness/atrophy, lethargy, coma, polyuria, excessive thirst, nausea vomiting, hypertension, ECG changes
Treatment – treat underlying cause

Magnesium
(normal range 0.7–1.0mmol/l)

- A major ICF cation closely related to potassium
- Essential in the function of many enzyme activities
- Has a depressant effect at the neural synapsis; also effects neuromuscular transmission and cardiovascular tone
- Renal function is central to magnesium homeostasis

Hypermagnesaemia
Renal failure; Excessive magnesium administration e.g. some antacids
Symptoms – Bradycardia, complete heart block, hypotension. In severe cases cardiac arrest and coma
Treatment – promotion of urinary output; IV fluid replacement and diuretics are used to 'flush out' excessive magnesium; calcium chloride via IV infusion (counteract effects of cardiovascular system)

Hypomagnesaemia
Malnourishment; diarrhoea/vomiting; increased renal excretion
Symptoms – muscular weakness/cramps; twitching and tremors; Cardiac arrhythmia (SVT, VT); tetany; convulsions and coma in severe cases
Treatment – IV replacement ICU admission (for continuous cardiac monitoring)); assessment of Kidney function prior to treatment; nutritional replacement

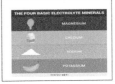

FIGURE 2.4 Electrolytes

PERIPHERAL VENOUS CANNULA (PVC)

Care of PVC site

➤ The PVC should be placed in the non-dominant hand/arm and is better positioned anywhere that will dislodge easily, e.g. the antecubital fossa.

➤ The gauge of the cannula should be appropriate to the type of fluid.

➤ Monitor the PVC site closely, e.g. when a bolus injection is given or an administration set is changed and when flow rates are checked or altered, for signs of complications.

➤ Monitor using the Visual Infusion Phlebitis score (VIP) score.

➤ If the VIP score is greater than or equal to 2 the PVC should be removed.

➤ Change the PVC dressing (when damp, coming off) using aseptic non touch technique (ANTT). Before dealing with dressing/PVC, wash hands and gain consent. The area should be cleaned with 2% chlorhexidine in 70% isopropyl alcohol (NICE 2014), moving from the catheter site outwards, providing it is compatible with the device (for children under 3 months use alcohol/sterile sodium chloride 0.9%). Allow to dry and then apply sterile dressing (epic3, Loveday *et al.* 2014)

➤ Flush the PVC before and after giving medication to check for and ensure patency but NOT if thrombo-embolism is suspected

➤ Change PVC when indicated.

(Cochrane Review, Ullman *et al.* 2015)

A cannula is a vascular device that is inserted into a peripheral or central blood vessel. Can be used for diagnostic blood sampling; invasive pressure monitoring; administration of intravenous fluids or drugs.

Removal of PVC

The PVC should be removed when no longer required or when indicated (e.g. showing signs of complications).

1. Wash and dry hands, put on appropriate protective clothing (non-sterile gloves and disposable apron).
2. Maintain hand hygiene.
3. Remove the dressing.
4. Gently remove the PVC.
5. Check the integrity of the PVC.
6. Immediately following the removal of the PVC, apply firm pressure with sterile gauze for 2–3 minutes or until bleeding has stopped. Care regarding patients with clotting disorders or on anticoagulant therapy.
7. If the site appears infected take and send a swab to microbiology.
8. Cover the puncture site with a sterile, adhesive dressing.
9. Documentation, and report any signs of complications.

Complications of PVC

- Catheter related blood stream infection
- Extravasation
- Haemorrhage
- Infiltration
- Phlebitis
- Blockage
- Thrombosis

VIP SCORE

Intravenous (IV) site appears healthy	**0**	No signs of phlebitis • Observe cannula
One of the following is evident: ▸ Slight pain near IV site ▸ Slight redness near IV site	**1**	Possible first signs of phlebitis • Observe cannula
Two of the following are evident: ▸ Pain near IV site ▸ Erythema ▸ Swelling	**2**	Early signs of phlebitis • Re-site cannula
All of the following are evident: ▸ Pain along path of cannula ▸ Erythema ▸ Induration	**3**	Medium stage of phlebitis • Re-site cannula • Consider treatment
All of the following are evident and extensive: ▸ Pain along path of cannula ▸ Erythema ▸ Induration ▸ Palpable venous cord	**4**	Advanced stage of phlebitis or start of thrombophlebitis • Re-site cannula • Consider treatment
All of the following are evident and extensive: ▸ Pain along path of cannula ▸ Erythema ▸ Induration ▸ Palpable venous cord ▸ Pyrexia	**5**	Advanced stage of thrombophlebitis • Initiate treatment • Re-site cannula

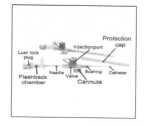

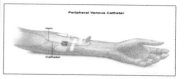

FIGURE 2.5 Peripheral venous cannula (PVC)

ADMINISTRATION OF INTRAVENOUS (IV) FLUIDS

1. Preparation

- Prepare work surface, have all equipment to hand
- Wash and dry hands
- Check identity of patient (name band and prescription chart), normally two checkers
- Give explanation to patient and gain consent (from patient or advocate)
- Check prescription adheres to the standards for prescribing
- Check name, strength, volume and expiry date of IV infusion against the prescription chart
- Check infusion fluid packaging is intact, inspect contents for signs of discolouration, cloudiness or particulate matter
- Select the correct administration set for the fluid to be administered (i.e. blood, blood products and electronic devices
- Check administration set expiry date

Hypotonic	Isotonic	Hypertonic
Used to replace electrolytes. Water moves into the cells via osmosis.	Most similar to body's plasma. Increases intravascular volume by fluid remaining in the extracellular compartment.	Has a higher concentration of solutes than the cell and will have a higher osmotic pressure outside the cell. This will cause water to be drawn from the cell.
Examples: 0.45% saline 0.18% saline	**Examples:** Ringers lactate 5% albumin 0.9% (normal) saline Hartmann's solution	**Examples:** Mannitol 20% albumin 3% saline

2. Setting up the IV fluid

- Open giving set packaging, being careful not to contaminate the ends of the tubing
- Close the roller clamp
- Using aseptic technique – remove the port protective covering of the fluid bag and remove the protective covering from the administration set
- Fully insert the spike of the administration set into the port of the fluid bag
- Hang the solution bag on the IV stand
- Squeeze the drip chamber gently until half full of solution
- Open the roller clamp to allow fluid to slowly fill the giving set
- Loosen/remove the cap at the end of the tubing (allow for the fluid to flow to the end of tubing)
- Tap tubing to help remove bubbles
- When there is no air – close roller clamp

3. Connecting to patient

- At all times maintain sterility of connection and tip of the administration set
- If an electronic device is used then this should be connected to the device
- Check identity of patient using the name band, prescription chart and infusion container
- Explain procedure to patient and gain consent
- Inspect the cannula site for signs of infection/blockage
- Wash hands
- Ensure that the cannula site is clean before administration
- Flush the cannula to ensure patency
- Connect the infusion to the IV cannula using non-touch technique
- Lock into position
- Secure tubing with tape
- Commence infusion and adjust flow rate (electronic device/drop calculation)
- Check patient for abnormal sensations/reactions
- Documentation (including fluid balance)
- Safe disposal of equipment
- Wash and dry hands

NICE (2017)

- Hospitals should have an IV fluid lead.
- Practitioners should be competent in assessing patient's fluid and electrolyte needs, prescribing and administrating fluids and monitoring patient's responses.
- A minimum of 24-hour IV fluid management plan.
- Events involving fluid mismanagement should be reported as critical incidents.

FIGURE 2.6 Intravenous infusion

INTRAVENOUS (IV) INFUSIONS

Route of administration

➢ Peripheral venous cannula (adult) (PVC)

➢ Central venous catheter (CVC)

➢ Skin tunnelled catheter (STC)

➢ Peripherally inserted central line (PICC)

Routine monitoring

❖ Pulse, blood pressure, capillary refill time
❖ Signs of pulmonary/peripheral oedema, postural hypotension
❖ Fluid balance chart
❖ Weight (if able)
❖ NEWS (NICE 2017)
❖ The cannula site for signs of inflammation / infection
❖ Check the patency of the IV fluid
❖ The type of fluid prescribed, rate of infusion
❖ Any anaphylactic reaction to the fluid from the patient

Major complications of IV therapy

- Cannula occlusion or damage
- Infiltration – leakage into tissues surrounding vein of non-irritant fluid
- Extravasation – infiltration of irritant fluid that cause tissue damage
- Thrombophlebitis
- Pulmonary/Air Embolism
- Bleeding/Haematoma
- Drug error
- Pain
- Shock/fluid overload
- Physical or chemical incompatibility/ interaction

Preventing infection

- Replace all tubing when vascular device is changed.
- All IV giving sets for peripheral and central use should be changed every 72 hours unless more frequently is indicated clinically.
- Replace blood and blood products IV giving sets every 12 hours and after every second unit of blood.
- Discard intermittent infusions sets immediately after use.

EPIC 3 Guidelines (Loveday *et al.* 2014)

Principles

IV fluid therapy should only be started if the patient's hydration needs cannot be met through oral or enteral routes.

Principles of IV fluid administration is for: Resuscitation, Routine maintenance, Replacement, Redistribution and Reassessment (5Rs).

A thorough assessment of the patient's fluid and electrolyte needs should occur

NICE (2017)

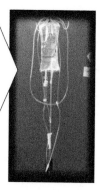

Calculating flow rates

$$\frac{\text{Volume of infusion (mls)} \times \text{number of drops per ml (from IV giving set)}}{\text{Time (minutes)}} = \text{flow rate (drops/minute)}$$

FIGURE 2.7 Starting an intravenous infusion

INFUSION DEVICES

Administration

The rationale for preparing and monitoring infusion sets and devices is to ensure patients are given the appropriate treatment, over the appropriate period and in a safe manner. There are a variety of sets dependent on the solution to be administered, e.g. crystalloids, blood. As equipment varies according to the manufacturer, the nurse must be familiar with the equipment used in the hospital/care environment. The 'drops' of fluid will vary in size (i.e. volume) and this will affect the rate at which they can be infused. In normal administration sets for clear fluids, each ml of fluid is determined as 20 drops. Ensure that the packaging is checked carefully as it will clearly indicate how many drops are in a ml, and this knowledge is necessary when calculating flow rates.

An infusion device is designed to accurately deliver measured amounts of fluid over a period of time (either intravenously or subcutaneously). It uses pressure to overcome resistance along the route of the infusion, pumping fluid from the infusion bag via an administration set and calculated volume to be delivered. It is designed to avoid **under/over infusion; metabolic disturbances; air embolism; phlebitis, toxic concentrations** or **concentrations below the therapeutic** dose.

With a gravity device the roller clamp is used to control the flow which is measured by counting the drops. With a gravity drip rate controller the desired flow rate is set in drops per minute and controlled by battery or valves.

Gravity flow infusion device

Consisting of an administration set containing a drip chamber and roller clamp. Usually measured by counting drops. Works on the principles of gravity to drive the infusion (good for infusions that do not have to be precise).

Patient controlled analgesia (PCA) pumps

These are syringe pumps that can deliver doses on demand (bolus dose). This type of pump is controlled by the patient.
They are categorised into 3 types:

1. *Basal rate* – a baseline rate is set but can be accompanied by intermittent doses controlled by the patient.
2. *Continuous* – designed for the patient who needs maximum pain relieve without the option of demand doses.
3. *Demand* – the drug is delivered by intermittent infusion and can be used alone or supplemented by the basal rate.

Volumetric pumps

Used for administration of large volumes of fluid. Calculates the volume delivered. Key features of these devices are that they can be battery as well as mains powered; able to overcome resistance to flow by increased release of pressure (not gravity); are capable of accurate delivery over a range of flow rates; have air in-line detectors, alarms.

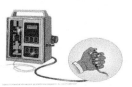

Syringe pump

Low-volume, high-accuracy device designed to infuse at low flow rates. The drive speed of the piston attached to the syringe driver controls the rate. Useful where small volumes of highly concentrated drugs need to be infused. Limited to the size of the syringe (60ml); mains and battery powered; easy to operate.

FIGURE 2.8 Infusion devices

ADMINISTRATION OF BLOOD TRANSFUSION

This procedure is considered to be an advanced role of the nurse, whereby the nurse has to be deemed competent though education, training and assessment. The primary person involved is a qualified nurse, but in some clinical settings a senior student could be the 'second checker'. In the case of paediatrics it is always the responsibility of two qualified nurses.

Pre-transfusion

- Make sure the blood is correctly and legibly prescribed.
- The patient/child should have a patent PVC access.
- Information must be provided to the patient/child/parent regarding the reasons for requiring the blood transfusion.

Pre-administration

- Check the prescription chart for any special requirements, e.g. any concurrent treatment such as diuretics.
- Make sure blood unit or bag is intact and has no leaks, discolouration or clumping.
- Take and record patient's baseline observations.
- Check the expiry date of component blood or blood product.
- Compatibility checks must be performed by **two people** at the bedside.
- Complete compatibility labels (these come with the blood product) and each nurse must sign them and add the date and the time.

Blood Types

Blood Type	Antigen on red blood cells	Antibodies in plasma	Can receive blood from	Can donate blood to
A	A	anti-B	O and A	A and AB
B	B	anti-A	O and B	B and AB
AB	A and B	neither	O, A, B, and AB	AB only
O	neither	anti-A and anti-B	O only	O, A, B, and AB

Labelled Blood Bag

Common adverse effects – adult

- Febrile
- Urticarial reaction (rash)
- Anaphylaxis
- Acute haemolytic reaction
- Bacterial contamination

Common adverse effects – child

- Febrile
- Urticarial rash (itchy rash)
- Anaphylaxis
- Increased diastolic BP (associated with febrile non-haemolytic transfusion reaction)
- febrile
- Pruritus/severe itching of the skin
- Nausea and vomiting
- Diarrhoea and stomach cramps

Administration of blood/blood products

- Remind patient of the reasons for the transfusion.
- Check the expiry date and that the blood/blood component will not expire during the transfusion episode (midnight of the expiry date as stated on the bag).
- Put on apron, wash hands and put on gloves.
- Blood should be transfused through a sterile administration set designed for the procedure. The set has a double chamber and must contain a 170-micron filter.
- Use prescribed 0.9% sodium chloride to prime the blood administration set.
- Attach the administration set to the venous access device, or if using a volumetric IV infusion pump, place the administration set in the infusion pump (as per manufacturer's guidelines). Set the rate and volume to be infused as stated on the fluid chart. Monitor throughout.
- The two staff members carrying out the patient identity checks and administering the blood must sign the fluid chart prescription, adding the date and time of the commencement of each transfusion.
- Vital signs of temperature, pulse and blood pressure must be recorded; check local policy for frequency, but normally are 5, 15, 30 and 60 minutes after infusion begins, then hourly until infusion completed, and then checked at the end of the transfusion.
- Patients must be in an area where they can be easily observed.
- The transfusion should be completed in less than 4 hours and the start and completion time should be recorded.
- Signs of a reaction include: pain at site of transfusion, loin pain, chest pain, breathing difficulties, anxiety, hypotension (more common in adults than children), collapse, rashes, rigors, or rise in temperature.
- A 1°C rise in temperature should be reported.
- In any of the above events the transfusion is stopped and the medical staff informed. The following actions may be taken but need to prescribed: loosen bedclothes/clothing; if prescribed, offer analgesia; if prescribed, offer antihistamines.
- Record the quantity of blood administered.
- Safely and appropriately dispose of equipment post-procedure.
- Keep empty blood bags.

FIGURE 2.9 Administration of blood

Activity: now test yourself

1   List five functions of water

2   Which is NOT a source of fluid loss?

Diarrhoea

Vomiting

Burns

Sweating

Bleeding

3   Indicate whether the following statements are true or false:

   a   A PVC should be changed every 72 h

   b   Extravasation is a complication of PVC

4   List five major complications of using IV infusions

5   Write the formula for calculating the flow rate of an IV infusion that is not being delivered via a delivery pump

Answers

1   Five from the following list:

Maintains and regulates body temperature

Helps maintain acid–base balance

Transports nutrients and oxygen to the cells

Dissolves minerals and other nutrients to make them accessible to the body

Lubricates joints, moistens tissues, i.e. in the eyes, mouth, nose

Protects body organs and tissues (acts as an insulator and shock absorber)

Excretion of metabolic waste products

Helps prevent constipation

2   *None – they are all sources of fluid loss*

3   a   False – *change when indicated*

   b   True

4   The list can include five of the following:

PVC occlusion or damage

Infiltration: leakage into tissues surrounding vein of non-irritant fluid

Extravasation: infiltration of irritant fluid that causes tissue damage

Thrombophlebitis

Pulmonary/air embolism

Bleeding/haematoma

Drug error

Pain

Shock/fluid overload

Physical or chemical incompatibility/interaction

5   **[Volume of infusion (ml) × number of drops per ml (from IV giving set)]/[Time (min) = flow rate (drops/min)]**

Reflection: ask yourself

1 What do I know that I did not know before?

2 What am I confused about now?

3 What areas do I need to focus on?

4 My action plan for further learning (make objectives SMART)

CHAPTER 3

Elimination and bowel care

Sheila Cunningham

Overview

As a fundamental need and physical activity, elimination is not only natural and essential but can also alter due to daily life stresses or behaviours. Bowel activity is complex and unique to individuals; however, it forms a key basic care need and one that nurses will definitely encounter on a daily basis.

Link to *Future Nurse Proficiencies* (NMC 2018)

Platform 4 Providing and evaluating care: specifically 4.6

Annexe B: Nursing procedures, Section 6: Use evidence-based, best practice approaches for meeting needs for care and support with bladder and bowel health, accurately assessing the person's capacity for independence and self-care and initiating appropriate interventions.

Expected knowledge

- Ability to describe the gastrointestinal tract segments and terms
- Anatomy of the exit orifices for elimination
- Personal hygiene around elimination episodes
- Infection control practices and precautions

Introduction

Bowel elimination is a sensitive issue, and providing effective care and management of issues or problems can be problematic due to this. The challenges can be minimised if the nurse seeks to respect patients' or clients' dignity during any encounter. There is a very wide range of what is considered 'normal'. The frequency of bowel actions and eliminations may range from several times per day to once per week. As a necessity, and as one of the activities of daily living, it occurs in every individual, yet is still embarrassing to discuss. Changes in elimination can result in anxiety and changes in behaviour as well as mood, which can be a challenge for people with learning difficulties, lack of language or confusion. This ought to be borne in mind when addressing elimination with patients or clients.

Content

Bowel assessment	Assisting with toilet or commode	Stoma care
Enemas	Suppositories	Stool assessment

Learning outcomes

- Outline normal defecation and challenges to this.
- Explain and describe nursing assistance with faeces elimination specifically:
- *Positioning for defecation*
- *Administration of an enema and suppositories*
- Assessment of faeces and recording
- Describe the key skills with administering enemas or suppositories

Key background

Elimination can be described as the removal of the waste products of digestion from the body human. These products will be in the form of urine or faeces (stool); the volume, amount, colour, frequency and consistency of these will depend on a variety of factors such as age, patient condition, lifestyle factors, pain and any prescribed medications. Normal stool output per day is around 150–200 g. The proximal colon defines the consistency and volume of delivery of contents to the rectum. Bowel frequency in a healthy person may vary between three times a day and three times a week. Stool consistency can vary and its production is influenced by gender, diet and health (RCN 2012). The purpose of assisting a patient with their elimination needs is to ensure that the patient is given prompt support in an ideal and appropriate setting. There are many reasons why a patient will need help with their elimination, such as frailty, cognitive impairment, poor mobility, injury and incontinence. Continence is the ability to voluntarily control emptying the bladder and bowels effectively in a socially acceptable and hygienic way. In the UK half a million people suffer with bowel control problems (Buckley and Lapitan 2009).

The gastrointestinal tract (and the lower end of the colon or bowel) is intimately connected with and controlled by the central nervous system – to be precise the autonomic path (sympathetic and parasympathetic). The neurological control of the bowel is the result of an intricate balance between the extrinsic and enteric nervous system, and the intestinal smooth muscle cells. Reflex pathways from the central nervous system to the intestine and colon both facilitate and inhibit gut motility.

Bowel care therefore has a wide scope and may include assessments and interventions of an intimate or seemingly invasive nature that must be carried out when there is a specific and adequate clinical need. Furthermore, as this is a body 'fluid', when providing bowel care healthcare professionals ought be aware of the need to follow standard infection prevention precautions.

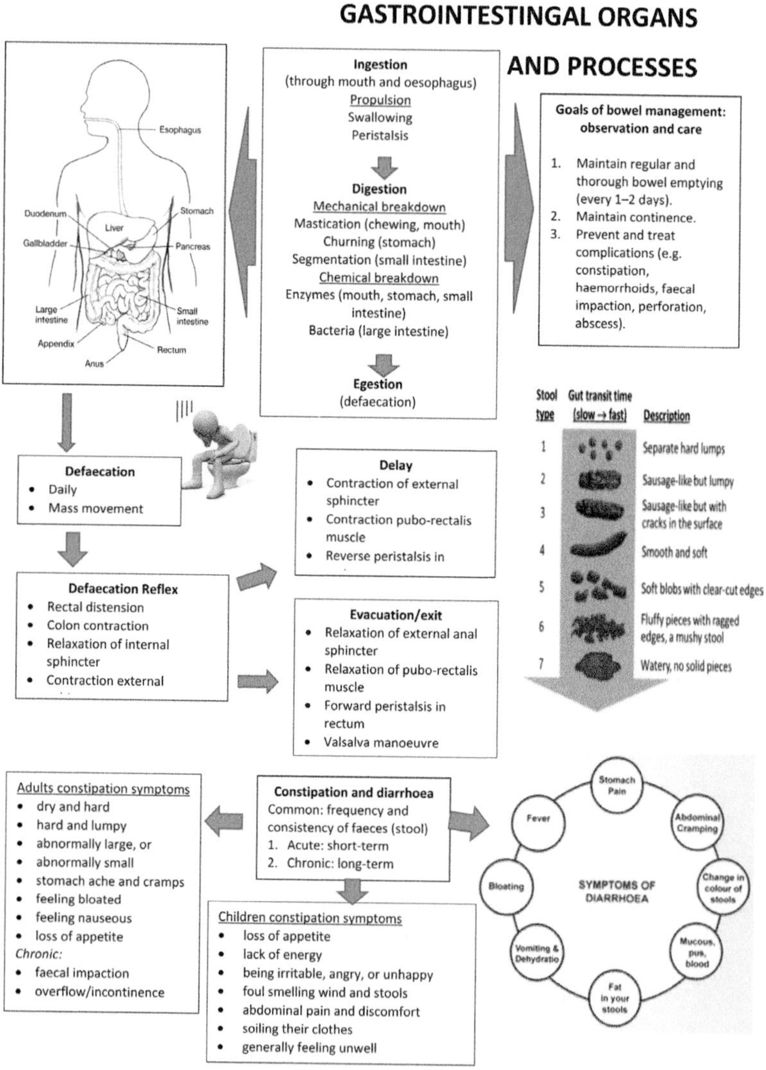
GASTROINTESTINGAL ORGANS
AND PROCESSES
Esophagus
Duodenum
Liver
Stomach
Gallbladder
Pancreas
Large intestine
Small intestine
Appendix
Rectum
Anus
Ingestion
(through mouth and oesophagus)
Propulsion
Swallowing
Peristalsis
Digestion
Mechanical breakdown
Mastication (chewing, mouth)
Churning (stomach)
Segmentation (small intestine)
Chemical breakdown
Enzymes (mouth, stomach, small intestine)
Bacteria (large intestine)
Egestion
(defaecation)
Goals of bowel management: observation and care
1. Maintain regular and thorough bowel emptying (every 1–2 days).
2. Maintain continence.
3. Prevent and treat complications (e.g. constipation, haemorrhoids, faecal impaction, perforation, abscess).
Defaecation
• Daily
• Mass movement
Defaecation Reflex
• Rectal distension
• Colon contraction
• Relaxation of internal sphincter
• Contraction external
Delay
• Contraction of external sphincter
• Contraction pubo-rectalis muscle
• Reverse peristalsis in
Evacuation/exit
• Relaxation of external anal sphincter
• Relaxation of pubo-rectalis muscle
• Forward peristalsis in rectum
• Valsalva manoeuvre
Stool type
Gut transit time (slow → fast)
Description
1 Separate hard lumps
2 Sausage-like but lumpy
3 Sausage-like but with cracks in the surface
4 Smooth and soft
5 Soft blobs with clear-cut edges
6 Fluffy pieces with ragged edges, a mushy stool
7 Watery, no solid pieces
Adults constipation symptoms
• dry and hard
• hard and lumpy
• abnormally large, or
• abnormally small
• stomach ache and cramps
• feeling bloated
• feeling nauseous
• loss of appetite
Chronic:
• faecal impaction
• overflow/incontinence
Constipation and diarrhoea
Common: frequency and consistency of faeces (stool)
1. Acute: short-term
2. Chronic: long-term
Children constipation symptoms
• loss of appetite
• lack of energy
• being irritable, angry, or unhappy
• foul smelling wind and stools
• abdominal pain and discomfort
• soiling their clothes
• generally feeling unwell
SYMPTOMS OF DIARRHOEA
Stomach Pain
Abdominal Cramping
Change in colour of stools
Mucous, pus, blood
Fat in your stools
Vomiting & Dehydratio
Bloating
Fever

FIGURE 3.1 Gastrointestinal tract and physiology

ASSISTING WITH ELIMINATION

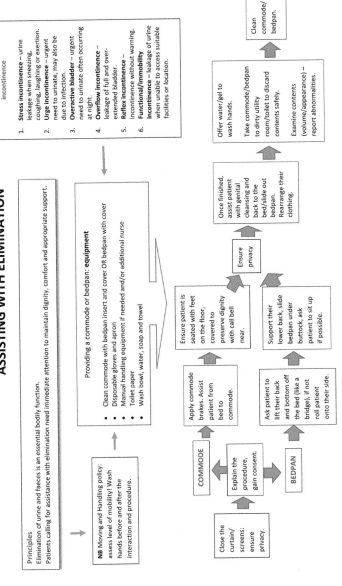

Principles

Elimination of urine and faeces is an essential bodily function.

Patients calling for assistance with elimination need immediate attention to maintain dignity, comfort and appropriate support.

Common types of urinary incontinence

1. **Stress incontinence** – urine leakage when sneezing, coughing, laughing or exertion.
2. **Urge incontinence** – urgent need to urinate, may also be due to infection.
3. **Overactive bladder** – urgent need to urinate often occurring at night.
4. **Overflow incontinence** – leakage of full and over-extended bladder.
5. **Reflex incontinence** – incontinence without warning.
6. **Functional/immobility incontinence** – leakage of urine when unable to access suitable facilities or location.

NB Moving and Handling policy: assess level of mobility! Wash hands before and after the interaction and procedure.

Providing a commode or bedpan: equipment

- Clean commode with bedpan insert and cover OR bedpan with cover
- Disposable gloves and apron
- Manual handling equipment if needed and/or additional nurse
- Toilet paper
- Wash bowl, water, soap and towel

Close the curtain/ screens: ensure privacy.

Explain the procedure, gain consent.

COMMODE

Apply commode brakes. Assist patient from bed to commode.

BEDPAN

Ask patient to lift their back and bottom off the bed (like a bridge), if not roll patient onto their side.

Support their lower back, slide bedpan under buttock, ask patient to sit up if possible.

Ensure patient is seated with feet on the floor, covered to preserve dignity with call bell near.

Ensure privacy

Once finished, assist patient with genital cleansing and back to the bed/slide out bedpan. Rearrange their clothing.

Offer water/gel to wash hands.

Take commode/bedpan to dirty utility room/toilet to discard contents safely.

Examine contents (volume/appearance) – report abnormalities.

Clean commode/ bedpan.

FIGURE 3.2 Assisting with elimination

ENABLING BOWEL ELIMINATION

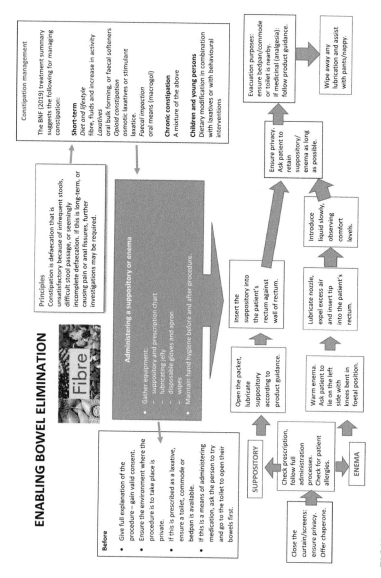

Constipation management

The BNF (2019) treatment summary suggests the following for managing constipation:

Short-term
Diet and lifestyle
fibre, fluids and increase in activity
Laxatives
oral bulk forming, or faecal softeners
Opioid constipation
osmotic laxatives or stimulant laxatice.
Faecal impaction
oral means (macrogol)

Chronic constipation
A mixture of the above

Children and young persons
Dietary modification in combination with laxatives or with behavioural interventions

Principles
Constipation is defaecation that is unsatisfactory because of infrequent stools, difficult stool passage, or seemingly incomplete defaecation. If this is long-term, or causing pain or anal fissures, further investigations may be required.

Administering a suppository or enema

- Gather equipment:
  - suppository and prescription chart
  - lubricating jelly
  - disposable gloves and apron
  - wipes
- Maintain hand hygiene before and after procedure.

Before

- Give full explanation of the procedure – gain valid consent.
- Ensure the environment where the procedure is to take place is private.
- If this is prescribed as a laxative, ensure a toilet, commode or bedpan is available.
- If this is a means of administering medication, ask the person to try and go to the toilet to open their bowels first.

Close the curtain/screens: ensure privacy. Offer chaperone.

SUPPOSITORY

Check prescription, follow full administration processes. Check for patient allergies.

ENEMA

Open the packet, lubricate suppository according to product guidance.

Warm enema. Ask patient to lie on the left side with knees bent in foetal position.

Insert the suppository into the patient's rectum against wall of rectum.

Lubricate nozzle, expel excess air and insert tip into the patient's rectum.

Introduce liquid slowly, observing comfort levels.

Ensure privacy. Ask patient to retain suppository/ enema as long as possible.

Evacuation purposes: ensure bedpan/commode or toilet is nearby. If medicinal (analgesia): follow product guidance.

Wipe away any lubrication and assist with pants/nappy.

FIGURE 3.3 Enabling bowel elimination

CHALLENGES WITH BOWEL ELIMINATION

Digital rectal examination (DRE)

A digital rectal examination (DRE) is an invasive procedure *not* routinely undertaken unless necessary, and then only by a suitably qualified and competent professionals (not student).

It may be a procedure seen in some areas, so its purpose should be understood. DRE can be used in the following circumstances to:

- establish the presence of faecal matter in the rectum (amount and consistency)
- ascertain anal tone and the ability to initiate a voluntary contraction, and to what degree
- establish anal and rectal sensation
- teach pelvic floor exercises
- assess anal pathology for the presence of foreign objects
- prior to giving any rectal medication, to establish the state of the rectum
- to establish the effects of rectal medication.

Haemorrhoids

These are a common problem, but the incidence data is unreliable and varies greatly.
Elimination may be affected, avoided or causing pain or discomfort, especially when sitting. Includes:

- pain during defaecation.
- itching or irritation around the anal region
- frank blood in stools or toilet paper
- swelling around the anus.

These need investigation, sensitivity and understanding and support during treatment. Treatment depends on the type, but may include:

- dietary fibre
- increased hydration
- weight management
- advice on straining to defecate
- if severe: surgery.

Chaperoning

It is important or recognise intimate examinations are embarrassing.
Patients may and can request a chaperone when undergoing any procedure or examination or treatment.
This ought to be recorded/documented.
Sensitive, patient-centred care and bowel care includes consideration to:

- consent
- age
- cultural/religious beliefs or restrictions on the patient (e.g. gender).

Causes of faecal incontinence

- Passive soiling – due to problems with anal sphincter pressure or damage
- Urgency and urge faecal incontinence (sphincter problems or obstetric trauma)
- Increased gut motility, e.g. infection, inflammatory bowel disease, irritable bowel syndrome, diet
- Rectal prolapse, fistula, haemorrhoids, neurological diseases, spinal cord injury, multiple sclerosis, spina bifida, dementia
- Lifestyle and environmental issues – poor toilet facilities, diet, dependence on carers for mobility and managing clothing
- Idiopathic or unknown cause.

Encopresis

- Also called faecal incontinence or soiling, is the repeated passing of stool (usually involuntarily) into clothing.
- It happens when impacted stool collects in the colon and rectum: the colon becomes too full and liquid stool leaks around the retained stool, staining underwear.
- May result in swelling (distention) of the bowels and loss of control over bowel movements.
- Often occurs after age 4, when the child has already learned to use a toilet.
- Often a symptom of chronic constipation or possible emotional issues.

Faecal incontinence

Most people acquire bowel control at a very young age and take the process very much for granted.
It is important to diagnose the specific problem and the cause or causes for the individual before treating (NICE 2007).

May be defined as follows:

- Passive soiling (liquid or solid) occurs when an individual is unaware of liquid or solid stool leaking from the anus; this may be after a bowel movement, or at any time (RCN 2019a).
- Anal incontinence is the involuntary loss of flatus, liquid or solid stool that is a social or a hygienic problem (Norton et al. 2010).

FIGURE 3.4 Challenges with elimination processes

What is a stoma?

- An opening on the abdomen – either your digestive or urinary system, to allow waste (urine or faeces) to be diverted out of the body.
- It looks like a small, pinkish, circular piece of flesh that is sewn to your body.
- It may lie fairly flat to the body or protrude out.
- Over the top of your stoma a pouch is worn which can either be closed or have an opening at the bottom.
- A stoma has no nerve endings so there is no pain sensation.

Why have a stoma?

- May be temporary or permanent.
- To cure or relieve disorders such as:
- bowel cancer, bladder cancer, inflammatory bowel disease (Crohn's disease or ulcerative colitis), diverticulitis or an obstruction to the bladder or bowel.

Stoma care

To maintain a healthy stoma and surrounding skin:

1. Observe colour of the stoma – pink, not overly oedematous.
2. Observe excretion material – if faeces, consistency and volume; if urine, colour and clarity.
3. Observe appliance – position, intact, draining.
4. Observe skin integrity around stoma – cleansing with dry wipes and water, no special solutions required (and may be damaging).

Changing a stoma bag

Prepare equipment needed including stoma bag, wipes, water, stoma template and waste bags.

Procedure summary:

1. *Encourage patient to do this and if unable to show them the procedure stages.*
2. Explain to patient, gaining consent.
3. Maintain hand hygiene at all stages.
4. If drainable, drain bag and dispose.
5. Protect patient clothing.
6. Peel back adhesive connecting pouch to skin gently and discard.
7. Wash stoma (water).
8. Observe skin and stoma.
9. Prepare stoma flange (sticks to skin and pouch to position it).
10. Using template cut correct size opening on flange.
11. Gently press into place.
12. Attach stoma bag – check for leakage.
13. Ensure patient is comfortable and document the stoma observations and task.

← STOMA CARE →

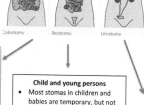

Colostomy   Ileostomy   Urostomy

Adults with dementia or confusion and stomas

Teaching a person with dementia how to care for their stoma is not possible in all cases, but where it is possible, attempts should be made to encourage them.

1. Consider surroundings (familiarity).
2. Break stages down and repeat.
3. Check for other issues impacting selfcare, e.g. hearing loss.
4. Reduce anxiety – do procedure in front of a mirror so patient can see themselves, making it part of other routines, e.g. brushing teeth.
5. Consider appliance choice, to minimise distress of changing bags (i.e. one- or two-piece bags).

Child and young persons

- Most stomas in children and babies are temporary, but not all.
- Reassure parent this is not a rare occurrence.
- Parent care for small children's stomas (see box right).
- Teenagers may have added anxieties: body image, clothing, being different, avoiding intimacy or relationships, body odours. Resources address these issues, as do supportive professionals, for example blogs and support groups in UK and Scotland (see www.colostomyUK.org).

FIGURE 3.5 Stoma care

Activity: now test yourself

1 How many phases are there to defecation?

2 Constipation can occur due a number of issues; which of the following do NOT cause constipation?

   a Exercise

   b Diet

   c Environmental pollution

   d Hydration

   e Stress or anxiety

3 What part of the nervous system is the colon enervated by?

4 Which of the following is true:

   a The sympathetic nervous system promotes movements relating to the bowel

   b The parasympathetic nervous system inhibits movements relating to the bowel

   c Peristalsis is the contractions of circular and longitudinal muscles of the intestine and occurs every 3–12 minutes

   d Haemorrhoids are arteries in the rectum that become abnormally distended

5 What is the term used to describe the technique of 'bearing down' when passing a bowel movement?

   a Haemorrhoids

   b Defecation

   c Valsalva's manoeuvre

   d Bowel elimination

Answers

1   There are two phases: defecation reflex (filling of lower colon, which is involuntary) and evacuation (exit, which is a voluntary phase).

2   c   Although it may cause changes to bowel habits, there is no known correlation to constipation; however, it may be that some pollutants will cause gastrointestinal changes, e.g. lead pollution.

3   The autonomic nervous system: parasympathetic and sympathetic

4   The correct answer is c

   Sympathetic nervous system inhibits bowel movements

   Parasympathetic nervous system relaxes the body and promotes bowel movements

   Haemorrhoids are related to the VEINS of the rectum becoming abnormally distended

5   Correct answer is c

   Defecation is normally assisted by taking a deep breath and trying to expel this air against a closed glottis (Valsalva's manoeuvre). This contraction of expiratory chest muscles, diaphragm and abdominal wall muscles exerts pressure on the digestive tract and enables elimination from the large intestine.

Reflection: ask yourself

1   What do I know now that I didn't know before?

2   What am I confused/unclear about?

3   What areas do I need to focus on?

4   My action plan for further learning (make objectives SMART)

CHAPTER 4

Renal function and care

Sheila Cunningham

Overview

Urinary elimination is a key body function and a subject that nurses ought to understand and address sensitivity with people who may have concerns about it. The process of control of urinary elimination or micturition occurs early in development around two years of age. However, this can vary somewhat. Similar to bowel elimination, it is a topic that can potentially be very embarrassing, especially with people who have altered elimination processes due to physical, psychological or emotional issues.

Link to *Future Nurse Proficiencies* (NMC 2018)

Platform 4 Providing and evaluating care: specifically 4.6

Skills annexe B, part 1: Procedures for assessing people's needs for person-centred care. Specifically 2.9: collect and observe sputum, urine, stool and vomit specimens, undertaking routine analysis and interpreting findings. 6.1 and 6.2: observe and assess level of urinary and bowel continence to determine the need for support and intervention assisting with toileting. 6.2: select and use appropriate continence products; insert, manage and remove catheters for all genders; and assist with self-catheterisation when required.

Expected knowledge

a Structure of the kidney and blood filtration to form urine
b Fluid balance and urine volumes produced daily

Introduction

The average adult passes about 1.5 litres of urine a day and depends on this urination to rid the body of organic waste products. For children this varies depending on diet, hydration, atmospheric temperature and activity. In general, if urine output is to be measured, it is monitored hourly and based on body weight. In general this is identified as:

- Neonate 2–3 ml/kg per h
- Infant 2 ml/kg per h
- Child 1– 2 ml/kg per h
- Adults or adolescents: approximately 0.5–1 ml/kg per h (Willock and Jewkes 2000)

The waste is produced as a result of cell metabolism, with the final composition of urine reflecting the internal status of the body (hydration, metabolism, etc.); it results from the filtration, absorption and secretion activities of the nephrons. Urine is an aqueous solution of approximately 95% water. Other constituents include urea, chloride, sodium, potassium, creatinine and other dissolved ions, and inorganic and organic compounds, which are eliminated depending on the need and status of the body.

Dehydration is a condition that can occur with excess loss of water and other body fluids. Dehydration results from decreased intake, increased output (renal, gastrointestinal or insensible losses), a shift of fluid (e.g. ascites, effusions) or capillary leak of fluid (e.g. burns and sepsis). Children and elderly or confused people are particularly susceptible to dehydration. However, dehydration aside, monitoring urine output is key, as is monitoring the constituents of the urine, and the patterns of and issues with elimination

Content

Micturition	Continence	Incontinence
Catheterisation	Urinalysis	

Learning outcomes

- Explain micturition and connection to voluntary bladder control
- Define elimination and continence
- Explain and describe nursing assistance with urine elimination specifically:
  - *Bladder training*
  - *Offering bedpans*
  - *Catheterisation*
- Outline the process and purpose of urinalysis

Key background

The process of elimination from the bladder is termed 'micturition' or 'voiding', and is both a voluntary and an involuntary action. It is voluntary in the sense that control of where and when to empty the bladder occurs at around the age of two years. This is termed 'continence'. The bladder does not have an infinite capacity and thus there are periods when the bladder will empty because it is too full despite the person not wishing to. Furthermore there are conditions and factors that alter the process of urinary elimination and lead to a situation of lack of control or incontinence. There are various types of alterations to urinary elimination termed 'incontinence' types, which have varied causes from nerve damage to pelvic floor muscle weakness or infection. It is estimated that there may be as many as three million people in the UK with urinary incontinence, of whom 60–80% have never sought medical advice for their condition with 35% viewing it simply as part of the ageing process (British Association of Urological Surgeons [BAUS] 2019). Furthermore, it is identified that conservative treatment (diet, weight management, pelvic floor exercises, etc.) can be successful in improving most forms of incontinence, so the patient or client has control and power to assist themselves with their own quality of life.

URINARY TRACT AND RENAL FUNCTION

Hydrated

Dehydrated

Extremely
Dehydrated
(consult a doctor)

Urinary tract
Kidneys
Ureters (tubes)
Bladder
Urethra

Urine (filtrate in nephron)
Ultrafiltration (*Bowman's capsule*)
Reabsorption (*proximal convoluted tubule*)
Water reabsorption (*Loop of Henle*)
Secretion and reabsorption
Adjustment (*distal convoluted tubule*)

Excretion (micturition)
Bladder reservoir
External ejection

Functions of Renal System

1. Removing waste products
2. Storing and eliminating urine
3. Regulation:
   - Blood volume and pressure regulation (renin-angiotensin, aldosterone hormones)
   - Erythrocyte regulation (erythropoietin hormone)
   - pH and acidity

Urine is a clear amber liquid comprising 95% water and 5% solids.

Wastes from metabolism (ammonia, uric acid, salts hormones etc.) affect the colour.

NO glucose of blood in healthy urine.

Volume

Varies with hydration, on average 1500 to 2000ml/day.
Urine is darker on waking compared to later in the day/before bedtime.
Problems in volume (frequency, small amounts, etc.) are investigated further.

Symptoms of UTI

Uncontrollable/frequent urge to urinate
Burning sensation on urination
Strong- or foul-smelling urine
Blood visible in urine
Fever
Pain in lower abdomen, lower back
Nausea and/or vomiting
Extreme cases: confusion

Causes of a cloudy urine

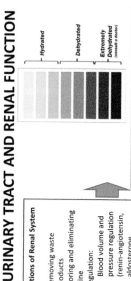

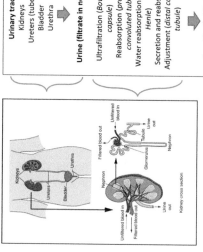

- Dehydration
- Pregnancy
- Vaginitis
- Kidney stones
- Sexually transmitted infections (STIs)
- Diabetes mellitus
- Urinary tract infections (UTIs)

FIGURE 4.1 Urinary tract and renal

MICTURITION AND CONTROL

Micturition

Micturition (urination) is the process of urine excretion from the urinary bladder.

Most of the time, the bladder (detrusor muscle) is used to store urine. The ability to voluntarily control micturition develops from 2 years as the nervous system develops.

Micturition mechanism

Micturition cycle occurs in two phases: a filling phase and an emptying phase, and is under voluntary and involuntary control.

Passing of urine is under parasympathetic control.

- During rest the bladder fills and the internal sphincter is closed (muscle keeps urine inside).
- At 450–500ml signals ascend, then descending signals contract the detrusor muscle and increase bladder pressure and the internal urethral sphincter relaxes. Finally, a voluntary contraction of the external urethral sphincter allows for the passing of urine.
- In the female, urination is assisted by gravity, while in the male contractions and squeezing along the length of the penis help to expel all of the urine.

Bladder training in adults

Occurs for a variety of reasons, e.g. following stroke. Can try the *One step at a time* approach (see lower left), or the following:

- Regular visit of the toilet with assistance if mobility is compromised
- Attending to timing and cues of bladder filling (prompting to void)
- Pelvic floor exercises
- Manipulation of clothing for access
- Personal hygiene and self-cleansing

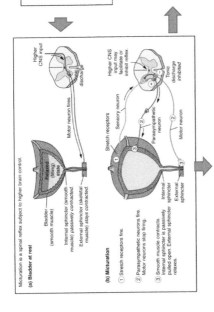

Micturition is a spinal reflex subject to higher brain control.

(a) Bladder at rest

Bladder (smooth muscle) – Relaxed (filling) state

Internal sphincter (smooth muscle) passively contracted.

External sphincter (skeletal muscle) stays contracted.

Higher CNS input

Motor neuron fires

Tonic discharge

(b) Micturition

① Stretch receptors fire.

② Parasympathetic neurons fire. Motor neurons stop firing.

③ Smooth muscle contracts. Internal sphincter is passively pulled open. External sphincter relaxes.

Higher CNS input may facilitate or inhibit reflex

Stretch receptors

Sensory neuron

Parasympathetic neuron

Motor neuron

Internal sphincter

External sphincter

Tonic discharge inhibited

Developing continence (in children)

Assess child for readiness and ability to 'hold on' and 'void', then aim for this approach: *One step at a time* (CFA 2010):

Step 1: Set the scene, location, time of day, sensation of wet/dry.

Step 2: Developing physical skills – sitting on toilet, puling pants up and down, washing hands.

Step 3: Raising awareness – how long the child can stay dry, move child out of disposable nappies/pants into washable underwear.

Step 4: Using the toilet and wiping own bottom.

Step 5: Night-time control eventually – if problematic may need support form a continence service/expert.

FIGURE 4.2 Micturition and control

CATHETER CARE REVIEW AND FOLLOW UP

Catheter care equipment review includes:
- Catheter size and length (especially if becoming ambulant)
- Catheter material
- Balloon size (should be 10ml, unless following prostatic surgery)
- There is a clear rationale for not using a catheter valve, and consequences
- Drainage bag capacity (day and night)
- Complications relating to wearing products or accidental disconnection
- Supply issues, stock levels and safe storage
- Correct emptying, changing and disposal techniques are used

Catheter sizes

THREE lengths but also different diameters (gauges):
- Paediatric: 30cm length and 6–10 CH gauge (narrow)
- Standard: 43cm length and 12–16 CH (mid-range)
- Female: 20–25cm and 12–14 CH gauge (*NOT to be used for males due to longer urethra*)

May also be wider for urine with solutes/clots etc. (up to 24 CH).

Vulnerable patients – catheter related problems

Anyone with a catheter is vulnerable, however some groups have further increased risk when having an indwelling urinary catheter:
- People in poor health and clustered into groups, e.g. in care homes or residential places.
- Orthopaedic patients, due to mobility issues and health status.
- Emergency areas – if catheter is inserted during lifesaving treatment it may be with compromised aseptic approach.
- Very young and confused – catheters are an irritant and maybe soiled or pulled, creating trauma.
- Those with poor hygiene or attention to catheter care.

Review of catheter care

Periodic review is needed including the following:
- A review of the patient urinary catheter passport, if used.
- A patient assessment: ongoing need for the urinary catheter and possible alternative methods.
- Documented rationale and plan for the continuing use of a urinary catheter.
- The patient's overall health status (conditions, medications and allergies.) including bladder health.
- The psychological impacts of catheterisation, on employment and home life.
- Review the patient's understanding and compliance with their catheter care.
- Review frequency of the catheter equipment and systems used and if need changing.
- Patient's hygiene practices around the catheter entry points: washing and care with meatus or perineum (special care with males' foreskin to avoid paraphimosis).
- Review the patient's daily fluid balance (in/out).
- Review the patient's bowel activity and relationship to the catheter function.
- Review the patient's confidence and capability to care independently for their catheter.

Bladder irrigation, installation and washouts

These do not prevent catheter-associated infection.

Regular use can lead to increased risk if the sterile closed drainage system is repeatedly broken.

In considering the use of washouts/maintenance solutions, there must be evidence of an individualised assessment, and the clinical indication for use must be recorded.

Bladder washouts

These involve flushing the bladder with sterile normal saline to remove clots, debris or mucus.

Considerations are shown in the next three boxes.

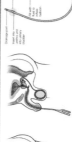

Why?

Best practice: small sequential volumes are more effective than a single larger volume.

There is a high risk of infection.

Caution

A clear, documented clinical rationale for using bladder washouts.

Irrigation used is sterile pre-filled administration set.

How?

Bladder washouts should be administered using gravity rather than direct pressure to avoid tissue trauma.

If in doubt ASK

FIGURE 4.3 Catheters

URINE SPECIMENS

MSU (Adults)

Instructions:
- Wash hands and genitals prior to taking sample.
- *WOMEN* – hold open the labia (entrance to the vagina).
  MEN – Pull back the foreskin.
- Pass some urine into the toilet (20–30 ml), then without stopping the flow of urine, catch some urine in the sterile bottle/container provided.
- Finish passing the rest of the stream of urine in the toilet.
- There is no need to fill the bottle to the top, any amount will enable testing.
- Care is needed to avoid touching any part of the genitals with the bottle/container, as this increases the risk of contamination.
- Put the cap back the sample bottle/container.
- Ensure the bottle/container is LABELLED immediately, including name and date of birth. This prevents the sample becoming misplaced from the requesting form when being sent to the laboratory.

Why take a specimen?
A urinalysis or midstream specimen of urine (**MSU**) is tested to look for infection.

Symptoms of a urine infection can include pain when passing urine or passing urine frequently.

Symptoms are not always typical, particularly in children and elderly.

Clean catch (children and babies)
It can be difficult to get a pure MSU sample from children and babies, so a 'clean catch' is an option. The following points are suggestions:

YOUNG CHILDREN
Be ready with the bottle open as the child passes urine, do not touch the open rim of the bottle with fingers, as this could contaminate the sample with bacteria.
BABIES
1. A special absorbent pad is placed into the nappy to absorb urine.
2. If no pad is available, take off the nappy about one hour after feed. Tap very gently with a finger just above the pubic bone. Often within about 5 minutes of doing this the baby will pass urine. Ensure catch bottle is ready.

Label with name and date of birth

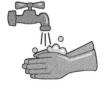

Clinical guidelines: preventing infection
Clinical guidance (NICE 2012) states that a catheter specimen of urine must be obtained via the sampling port only, using an aseptic technique.

Almost all drainage bags on the UK health products market have an integral sampling port for specimen collection. Any that do not should be avoided. Many ports also allow for needleless sampling to reduce the risk of a sharps injury.

Catheter specimen of urine (CSU)
- Explain the procedure to the patient and gain valid consent.
- Wash hands thoroughly and wear disposable gloves.
- Observe catheter tubing for urine, if none visible clamp the tubing just below the sampling port (NOT the catheter).
- Clean the sample port with an alcohol-impregnated swab and allow to dry.
- In needleless collection, insert the syringe into the port (follow manufacturer's instructions). Aspirate urine and remove the syringe.
- In needle collection, insert the needle into the port at a 45° angle. Aspirate urine and remove the needle from port.
- Label the specimen as identified under MSU guidance, seal securely in specimen bag, wash hands.

Supra pubic catheter specimen
Follows the same principles for CSU.

FIGURE 4.4 Urine specimens

URINALYSIS

What is it?

- Urine is an external indicator of the state and functioning of the of the human body internally.
- Routine screening may be offered or uses to determine the status (e.g. hydration, nutrient status).

In general there are three indications:
- Screening – for systemic disease such as diabetes mellitus, or renal disease, or if there is a concern such as blood evident in the urine.
- Diagnosis – to confirm or exclude suspected conditions, e.g. urinary infections.
- Monitor progress of a condition or treatment, such as diabetes mellitus or urinary infections.

A complete urinalysis consists of three distinct testing phases:
1. Visual examination – colour and clarity
2. Chemical examination (dip stick) – up to 9 substances (bilirubin, white cells, blood etc.) that provide valuable information
3. Microscopic examination – to identify cells, casts, crystals and any bacteria present

Process

- Simple test using 'dip sticks', or more complex involving sending a urine sample to a laboratory for testing.
- Initial analysis of volume and physical characteristics, then chemical and microscopic properties.

Findings from urinalysis might include:

- **Glucose** – not normally found in urine, might be suggestive of diabetes or poor diet.
- **Protein** – not normally found in urine, may indicate infection.
- **White blood cells** – not normally in urine, may indicate kidney or urine infections.
- **Blood** – not usually found in urine, points to kidney disease, kidney stones, tumours, infections and trauma.
- **Bilirubin** – pigment from destruction of red blood cells, high levels may indicate effective liver function.
- **Ketones** – metabolic waste from fat breakdown, seen in reducing diets or diabetes mellitus.
- **Specific gravity** – urine concentration/density.
- **Urobilinogen** – high levels may suggest liver disease and low levels might indicate gallstones.

Characteristics of urine

- Clear (unless freshly voided, and may be cloudy initially).
- Pale to deep yellow: the colour may alter due to diet (beetroot, vitamin B) or illness (infection).
- Slightly acidic (pH6, but varies depending on diet: vegetarian results in more alkaline urine and omnivore a more acidic urine) – *be warned, if a sample is not fresh the pH changes (increases due to nitrogen degrading)*.
- Density (specific gravity) varies depending on hydration (from 1.000, i.e. same as pure water, to 1.035, or more concentrated).
- Odour characteristically 'aromatic', not foul.

Dipstick (reagent) test

This is the most common. Dipsticks are strips impregnated with chemical reactive pads designed to detect the presence or amount of certain substances present in the urine.

Procedure:
- Prepare equipment (urine sample, dipsticks, gloves, appropriate waste bin).
- Check expiry date of the dipsticks.
- Wash hands and don gloves.
- Dip the strips into the urine, fully immerse then withdraw the strips and tap gently on the side of the urine container to remove excess urine.
- Ensure the reagent pads are not leaking/merging (invalidates results).
- Hold the strip flat.
- Wait the required time interval.
- Compare the strip colour pads to the colour chart.
- Document and report results.

FIGURE 4.5 Urinalysis

Activity: now test yourself

1   Normal urine primarily consists of:

    a   Water, protein and sodium

    b   Water, urea and protein

    c   Water, urea and chloride

    d   Water, urea and glucose

2   If left standing at room temperature, a urine sample pH will:

    a   Decrease

    b   Increase

    c   Remain the same

    d   Change depending on bacterial concentration

3   One type of incontinence is stress incontinence. Stress urinary incontinence means that a person releases urine when they cough, sneeze, or do things such as bend down, lift or walk.

    a   True

    b   False

4   The catheter urinary collection bag should be positioned so that urine is always flowing:

    a   Sideways

    b   Upwards

    c   Downwards

    d   Any direction is fine

5 What are the typical signs and symptoms of a urinary tract infection?

   a   Excessive urine output, burning and clear yellow urine

   b   Fever greater than 38°C, blood in the urine and offensive urine odour

   c   Change in mental status, decreased urine output and bladder spasms

   d   Sediment in the urine, redness around the catheter insertion site and urine leakage

Answers

1 c   Water, urea and chloride

Urine will not contain protein or glucose – it is unlikely to have chloride in it, but is usually found to have sodium. The balance of sodium and water within the body is maintained to ensure adequate hydration and electrolytes for normal cell functioning, but can also be excreted.

2 a   Decrease

This is due to the breakdown of nitrogenous elements within the urine and this lowers the pH giving an inaccurate reading.

3 a   True

The leakage of urine on exertion to the abdominal walls and pelvic floor is known as 'stress' because it stresses the muscles and thus fails to retain urine during these behaviours.

4 c   Downwards

This is critical if urine is left to flow backwards because it can re-enter the bladder and cause stasis and risk of infection; this is compounded by the catheter, which increases the risk of infection.

5 b   Fever greater than 38°C, blood in the urine and offensive urine odour

There are aspects of all the answers that are correct; however, the fully correct one is b because this features all the signs of inflammatory changes and irritation, hence the blood, smell (from bacteria present) and the pain due to inflammation.

Reflection: ask yourself

1 What do I know now that I didn't know before?

2 What am I confused/unclear about?

3 What areas do I need to focus on?

4 Action plan for further learning (make the objectives SMART)

Bibliography

British Association of Urological Surgeons (BAUS) (2019) *Incontinence of urine* (online). Available at: www.baus.org.uk/patients/conditions/5/incontinence_of_urine (accessed 20 May 2019).

Buckley, B.S. and Lapitan, M.C.M. (2009) Prevalence of urinary and faecal incontinence and nocturnal enuresis and attitudes to treatment and help-seeking amongst a community-based representative sample of adults in the United Kingdom. *International Journal of Clinical Practice* **63**: 568–573.

Care Quality Commission (2011) *Dignity and Nutrition Inspection Programme: National Overview.* London: Care Quality Commission.

Continence Foundation of Australia (CFA) (2010) *One Step at a Time: A parent's guide to toilet skills for children with special needs.* Heidelberg, VIC: Victoria Continence Resource Centre.

Gitlin, M. (2016) Lithium side effects and toxicity: Prevalence and management strategies. *International Journal for Bipolar Disorders* **4**: 27.

Hodgkinson, B., Evans, D. and Wood, J. (2003) Maintaining oral hydration in older adults: A systematic review. *International Journal of Nursing Practice* **9**:s19–s28.

Loveday, H.P., Wilson, J.A., Pratt, J.J. *et al.* (2014). epic3: National Evidence-Based Guidelines for Preventing Healthcare-Associated Infections in NHS Hospitals in England. *Journal of Hospital Infection* Jan, **86**(Suppl):s1–s70.

National Institute for Health and Care Excellence (NICE) (2006) *Nutrition Support in Adults: Oral nutrition support, enteral tube feeding and parenteral nutrition. NICE clinical guideline* [CG32]. London. NICE.

National Institute for Health and Care Excellence (NICE) (2007) *Faecal Incontinence in Adults: Management. NICE Clinical Guideline* [CG49]. London: NICE.

National Institute for Health and Care Excellence (NICE) (2012) *Quality Statement 4: Urinary catheters. NICE Clinical Guideline* [CG139]. Available at: www.nice.org.uk/guidance/cg139 (accessed 16 May 2019).

National Institute for Health and Care Excellence (NICE) (2014) *Infection Prevention and Control. NICE Clinical Guideline* [QS61]. London: NICE.

National Institute for Health and Care Excellence (NICE) (2017) *Intravenous Fluid Therapy in Adults in Hospital. NICE Clinical Guideline* [CG174]. London: NICE.

National Institute for Health and Care Excellence (NICE) (2019) *British National Formulary (BNF)*. London: NICE. Available at: https://bnf.nice. org.uk/treatment-summary/constipation.html (accessed 14 November 2019).

Norton, C., Whitehead, W.E., Bliss, D.Z., Harari, D. and Lang, J. (2010) Management of faecal incontinence in adults: Report from the 4th international consultation on incontinence. *Neurourology Urodynamics* **29**(1):199–206, DOI:10.1002/nau.20803.

Nursing and Midwifery Council (NMC) (2018) *Future Nurse Proficiencies*. London: NMC. Available at: www.nmc.org.uk/standards/standards-for-nurses/standards-of-proficiency-for-registered-nurses (accessed 1 May 19).

Royal College of Nursing (RCN) (2012) *Management of Lower Bowel Dysfunction*. London: RCN.

Royal College of Nursing (RCN) (2016) *Standards for Infusion Therapy*, 4th edn. London: RCN.

Royal College of Nursing (RCN) (2019a) *Bowel Care Management of Lower Bowel Dysfunction, including Digital Rectal Examination and Digital Removal of Faeces*. London: RCN.

Royal College of Nursing (RCN) (2019b) *Catheter Care: RCN Guidance for Health Care Professionals*. London: RCN.

Royal College of Nursing and National Patient Safety Agency (2007) *Water for Health. Hydration Best Practice Toolkit for Hospitals and Healthcare*. London: RCN/NPSA.

Thibodeau, G.A. and Patton. K.T. (2012) *Structure and Function of the Body*. 14th edition. St Louis, MO: Mosby.

Ullman, A.J., Cooke, M.L., Mitchell, M., Lin, F., New, K., Long, D.A., Mihala, G. and Rickard, C.M. (2015) Dressings and securement devices for central venous catheters (CVC). *Cochrane Database of Systematic Reviews* (9).

Webster, J., Osbourne, S., Rickard, S., Rickard, C.M. (2015) Clinically-indicated replacement versus routine replacement of peripheral venous catheters (Review). *Cochrane Database of Systematic Reviews* (8).

Wilcox, M. (2014) epic3: National evidence based guidelines for preventing healthcare associated infections in NHS hospitals in England. *Journal of Hospital Infection* **86**(Suppl 1):s1–s70.

World Health Organization (WHO) (2009) *WHO Guidelines on Hand Hygiene in Health Care*. Geneva: WHO. Available at: https://apps.who. int/iris/bitstream/handle/10665/44102/9789241597906_eng.pdf; jsessionid=09BB349AD9998F3342A3ED29D72116D9?sequence=1 (accessed 16 May 2019).

World Health Organization (WHO) (2017) *Protecting, Promoting and Supporting Breast Feeding in Facilities: Providing maternity and newborn services*. Geneva: WHO.

Index